The Yoga Custom: "Unveiling the Rich Tapestry of Yoga Customs"

Dolores E. Flint

Disclaimer

Table of contents

INTRODUCTION

Welcome to "The Yoga Custom." In this investigation of the ancient practice, we will go on a trip to discover the vast dimensions of yoga. Explore its historical roots, philosophical basis, and transforming potential for the mind, body, and soul. Allow the pages to lead you through the intricate tapestry of yoga traditions, providing insights on postures, breath control, meditation, and the yogic lifestyle. Join me in understanding how this time-honored custom can be easily integrated into the fabric of our modern lives to improve our well-being and spiritual connection. Within the pages of "The Yoga Custom," we explore the rich geography of yoga as more than a physical practice. It functions as a lighthouse, illuminating the way to self-discovery and overall well-being. As we embark on this journey, we'll trace the evolution of yoga from its ancient roots to its current relevance. In the following chapters, we'll look at the skill of asana, the mysteries of breath control through pranayama, and the transformational power of meditation and mindfulness. The yogic lifestyle, which includes nutrition, daily routines, and spiritual components, serves as a guide for achieving balance and harmony in all aspects of life. Beyond the mat, we look at how yoga fits into our modern lives. Relationships, stress management, and a larger understanding of yoga's purpose outside the mat become essential components of our investigation. This trip invites you to see yoga not just as a collection of physical exercises, but as a holistic philosophy for navigating the challenges of modern life.

Let us discover the ageless knowledge of "The Yoga Custom" together, promoting a deeper connection to oneself, others, and the world around us. May this journey inspire significant transformation, inviting you to incorporate yoga into the fabric of your unique existence.

The Foundations of Yoga

In "The Foundations of Yoga," we explore the essence and origins of this ancient practice. Explore the historical roots of yoga's evolution, as well as the philosophical principles that serve as its foundation. As we delve into these essential characteristics, we unravel the tapestry that connects yoga to its roots, laying the groundwork for our transforming journey through "The Yoga Custom." Yoga's foundation is a detailed investigation of its historical roots, which span thousands of years and are deeply rooted in various cultures. From ancient scriptures like the Vedas and Upanishads to classical yoga books like Patanjali's Yoga Sutras, we find the vast reservoir of wisdom that has fashioned yoga into the form it is today. Beyond history, the philosophical concepts of yoga lead practitioners on a transforming journey. Patanjali's concept of the Eight Limbs of Yoga provides a complete framework for self-realization. These limbs comprise ethical standards (yamas and niyamas), physical postures (asanas), breath control (pranayama), and meditation (dhyana), which are the foundation of a holistic yogic existence. As we create the platform for yoga, we see that it is more than just a physical exercise; it is a profound philosophy that strives to balance the mind, body, and spirit. This inquiry lays the groundwork for greater knowledge and embodiment of the yogic ideas found in "The Yoga Custom." At its core, yoga is a timeless journey that combines ancient knowledge and practical philosophy. Exploring the historical foundations reveals a tapestry woven through nations and civilizations, from the ancient Indus Valley to the yogic practices described in literature such as the Bhagavad Gita. This historical context deepens our understanding of yoga's continuity and flexibility over the millennia. Philosophically, yoga's basis is built on guiding concepts that go well beyond the physical postures that are typically associated with it. The Yamas and Niyamas, or ethical and moral principles, serve as the moral compass for a yogic lifestyle. These principles inspire practitioners to develop characteristics including honesty, nonviolence, contentment, and self-control. As we look at the foundations, the Eight Limbs of Yoga provide a thorough blueprint for personal development. These limbs bring practitioners toward a complete awareness of life, from physical postures (asanas) to breath control (pranayama), and finally to meditation (dhyana) that leads to self-realization (samadhi).

The essence of yoga is a multidimensional investigation that combines history, philosophy, and practical application. It acts as a guide for connecting one's inner self with the world, promoting not just physical well-being but also a fundamental sense of harmony and balance throughout human life. This comprehensive foundation lays the groundwork for the transforming journey contained inside "The Yoga Custom."

Ai. Yoga has ancient roots, dating back to the Indus Valley civilizations circa 2700 BCE. The earliest evidence comes from seals depicting figures in yoga poses, indicating a practice that combined physical, mental, and spiritual aspects. Yoga's journey continues during the Vedic period (1500-500 BCE), when sacred scriptures such as the Rigveda use the term "yoga." The Upanishads, which date back to roughly 800-200 BCE, offer philosophical ideas and investigate the unification of individual awareness with the universal. Patanjali's Yoga Sutras, compiled between 200 BCE and 200 CE, represent the crystallization of yogic philosophy. This foundational literature defines the Eight Limbs of Yoga and provides a step-by-step approach to self-realization. During the medieval period, other yogic systems evolved, including Hatha Yoga, which focuses on physical postures and breath control. Bhakti and Jnana Yoga lineages also thrived, adding to the rich tapestry of yoga practices. Yoga regained popularity in colonial India, thanks to people such as Swami Vivekananda, who introduced it to the West in the late nineteenth century. In the twentieth century, pioneers such as B.K.S. Iyengar and Pattabhi Jois helped to popularize various kinds of yoga around the world.

Understanding yoga's historical roots reveals a story of evolution, adaptation, and resilience, demonstrating its long-lasting relevance and transforming impact across cultures and time.

1. Yoga Through the Ages: Revealing Ancient Wisdom.

This book goes into the archeological evidence of yoga's roots, examining artifacts and ancient writings to get insight into the early practices of yoga in civilizations such as the Indus Valley and beyond.

2."Vedic Echoes: Tracing Yoga in the Vedas".

This book, which focuses on the Vedic period, studies the hymns and verses in the Rigveda, looking for subtle connections to yoga practices as well as the early philosophical foundations that laid the groundwork for later yogic traditions.

3."Upanishadic Wisdom: Yoga Unveiled".

Discover the profound lessons of the Upanishads, in which sages pondered the nature of reality and self. This book investigates how these intellectual inquiries paved the way for the spiritual qualities inherent in yoga.

4."Patanjali's Legacy: The Yoga Sutras Decoded".

This book provides an in-depth investigation of Patanjali's Yoga Sutras, breaking down each sutra to uncover the full system of ethics, postures, and meditation that has influenced modern yoga.

5."Yoga Renaissance: From Hatha to Modern Practices".

This book chronicles the history of Hatha Yoga from the medieval period to the current day, examining its emergence and growth into numerous modern versions. It looks at major figures who helped popularize yoga around the world.

6."Colonial Crossroads: Yoga in the 19th Century".

This book investigates the connection between colonialism and yoga, shedding insight into how encounters with the West shaped the perception and spread of yoga, particularly through people such as Swami Vivekananda.

7."Universal Gurus: Promoting Yoga in the 20th Century".

This book features notable yogis such as B.K.S. Iyengar, Pattabhi Jois, and others who were instrumental in bringing varied yoga approaches to the global arena and establishing the current landscape of yoga practice.

These volumes present a comprehensive narrative, unraveling yoga's historical origins spanning epochs and giving light to its many cultural, philosophical, and global elements.

ii.1. Yamas' Ethical Foundations

Investigate the ethical principles known as Yamas, which include ahimsa (nonviolence), satya (truthfulness), asteya (nonstealing), brahmacharya (celibacy or moderation), and aparigraha (non-attachment). These lead practitioners to virtuous and conscientious living.

2. Niyama: Personal Disciplines.
Explore the Niyamas, which include personal observances such as saucha (cleanliness), santosha (contentment), tapas (self-discipline), svadhyaya (self-study), and Ishvara

pranidhana (surrender to a higher power). These ideas promote internal strength and self-awareness.

3. Asanas are physical postures.

Understand the importance of physical postures (asanas) in yoga practice. Beyond the physical benefits, each posture promotes self-discovery, attention, and overall well-being.

4. Pranayama (Breath Control)

Learn about pranayama, the practice of using breath to cultivate life force energy. Learn several strategies for controlling and channeling the breath, which connects the physical body to the mind and spirit.

5. Meditation and Dhyana.

Dive into the transforming practice of meditation (dhyana). This section delves into several meditation practices, helping practitioners toward inner quiet and heightened awareness.

6. The Eight Limbs Of Yoga

Navigate the Eight Limbs of Yoga as described by Patanjali. These limbs provide a comprehensive path to spiritual progress, covering everything from ethical principles (yamas and niyamas) to physical postures (asanas), breath control (pranayama), and stages of meditation leading to self-realization (samadhi).

7. Karma & Bhakti Yoga

Learn the principles of Karma Yoga, which emphasizes altruistic action, and Bhakti Yoga, which focuses on devotion. These routes provide many ways for people to connect with the divine and develop a feeling of purpose.

As we investigate the theory and practices of yoga, we discover a comprehensive roadmap for balancing the physical, mental, and spiritual aspects of life. These fundamental elements act as a road map, promoting not just physical well-being but also a deep sense of purpose, inner serenity, and interconnectedness.

The physical practice of yoga, known as asanas, goes beyond simple poses to provide a transforming journey for the body, mind, and soul.

1. Standing poses:

Explore core poses like Tadasana (Mountain Pose) and the Warrior series, which provide strength, balance, and grounding. Standing poses provide a solid basis for physical practice.

2. Seated Poses: Practice seated postures like Sukhasana (Easy Pose) and Padmasana (Lotus Pose) to improve flexibility, hip opening, and mindfulness. Seated postures promote reflection and focus.

3. Inversions: Practice inversions like Headstand and Shoulderstand to increase strength, improve circulation, and focus, and gain a new viewpoint.

4. Backbends: Positions like Cobra and Bridge open the chest and heart, promoting emotional release, spinal flexibility, and better posture.

5. Forward Bends: Uttanasana (Forward Fold) helps stretch the spine and hamstrings while soothing the nervous system. They promote reflection and relaxation.

6. Twists: Twisting positions, such as Marichyasana, promote spinal flexibility and detoxification. Twists improve digestion and balance.

7. Balancing positions: Balancing positions like Tree Pose and Eagle Pose help improve focus, coordination, and stability. They encourage mindfulness and concentration.

Asanas are more than just physical exercises; they also serve as doorways to deeper self-awareness. Yoga is a physically demanding activity that promotes strength, flexibility, and balance. It also promotes attention, focus, and an interior journey. The interplay of breath and movement in each posture transforms into a moving meditation that promotes overall well-being. In "The Yoga Custom," the physical practice is explored as an important component of the larger tapestry of yogic concepts.

A. "Asanas: The Art of Postures" guides practitioners on a journey of self-discovery via the physical expressions of yoga. Each pose, or asana, serves as a canvas for developing strength, flexibility, and balance that extends beyond the physical world.

1. Standing Poses: Standing poses, such as the Mountain Pose (Tadasana) and Warrior series, provide practitioners with strength and stability. These earth-based postures serve as a solid basis for the practice.

2. Seated Poses: Seated asanas like Lotus Pose (Padmasana) and Easy Pose (Sukhasana) promote contemplation and flexibility. They encourage people to practice stillness, quiet their minds, and strengthen their connection with their inner selves.

3. Inversions: Inversions like Headstand (Sirsasana) and Shoulderstand (Sarvangasana) test gravity and provide a unique perspective. These postures promote circulation, vitality, and mental clarity.

4. Backbends: Backbends such as Cobra Pose (Bhujangasana) and Bridge Pose (Setu Bandhasana) help open the heart and promote emotional discharge. They encourage spinal flexibility and a feeling of expansiveness.

5. Forward Bending Asanas: Forward Fold (Uttanasana) focuses attention inward, stretching the spine and soothing the nervous system. They promote reflection and relaxation.

6. Twists: Twisting positions, such as Marichyasana, help cleanse the body and improve spinal mobility. Twists also represent the release of stress, which promotes a sense of rejuvenation.

7. Balancing Poses: Balancing positions, including Tree Pose (Vrikshasana) and Eagle Pose (Garudasana), offer more than just physical stability. They need attention, mindfulness, and the cultivation of inner balance.

Practitioners embark on a dynamic investigation of "Asanas: The Art of Postures," not only honing the physical body but also delving into the intricacies of breath, mindfulness, and the nuanced waltz between movement and quiet. This part unfolds as a canvas for self-expression and self-realization within the larger tapestry of yoga in "The Yoga Custom."

Ai. Standing poses are the cornerstone of yoga's physical practice, promoting strength, balance, and a deep connection to the ground. Learn about the creativity and benefits of key standing asanas:

1. Tadasana (Mountain Pose): Stand tall, feet hip-width apart, and ground through all portions of the foot. Tadasana rebalances the body, improves posture, and fosters a sense of stability and presence.

2. Virabhadrasana I (Warrior I): This pose strengthens the legs, extends the spine, and promotes courage and empowerment.

3. Virabhadrasana II (Warrior II): This position expands the hips and chest, increasing physical and mental energy. Warrior II fosters a solid foundation while encouraging focus and concentration.

4. Trikonasana (Triangle Pose): The body expands laterally, stretching along the sides. This asana increases balance, leg strength, and spinal flexibility.

5. Utthita Parsvakonasana (Extended Side Angle Pose): This deep side stretch with a balanced stance strengthens the legs, activates the core, and increases general body awareness.

6. Ardha Chandrasana (Half Moon Pose): This one-legged balance pose strengthens the ankles, thighs, and core while challenging stability. It also broadens the chest and promotes a sensation of expansiveness.

7. Vrikshasana (Tree Pose): Balancing on one leg, this pose improves concentration, balance, and posture. It represents rootedness and growth, promoting a link between body and mind.

These standing postures are more than just physical exercises; they allow practitioners to embody attributes such as strength, attention, and grounding. Incorporating these into a daily practice serves as a firm foundation for the more in-depth investigation of yoga in "The Yoga Custom."

ii. Seated yoga poses promote introspection, flexibility, and a deep connection with one's inner self. Discover the grace and advantages of essential sitting asanas:

1. Sukhasana (easy pose):

Sukhasana, a basic cross-legged pose, promotes ease and attention. It is a basic stance for meditation and pranayama that promotes a grounded and calm mood.

2. Padmasana (Lotus Pose) represents balance and purity. It is a more advanced seated pose that helps spine alignment, calms the mind, and improves focus during meditation.

3. Baddha Konasana (Bound Angle Pose), also known as Butterfly Pose, helps expand the hips and groins. It is a mild stretch that promotes flexibility and acts as a warm-up for deeper seated positions.

4. Janu Sirsasana (Head-to-Knee Forward Bend): This pose stretches the spine and hamstrings and promotes contemplation. Janu Sirsasana promotes submission and relieves tension.

5. Ardha Matsyendrasana (Half Lord of the Fishes Pose): This seated twist improves spine flexibility and promotes detoxification. This pose stimulates the digestive organs and promotes a feeling of regeneration.

6. Siddhasana (Adept's stance): This meditative stance aligns the spine and allows for long periods of seated meditation. It creates a relaxed and concentrated state of mind.

7. Virasana (Hero Pose): Sit on the shins to extend the thighs and ankles. It is a stance that promotes perfect alignment, fosters humility, and serves as a foundation for meditation.

Seated positions in yoga are about more than just flexibility; they also allow for contemplation, tranquility, and a connection to one's inner self. Incorporating these positions into practice helps to maintain a balance between the grounded quality of sitting and the expanding aspects of the mind and spirit in "The Yoga Custom."

iii. Inversions in yoga reverse the typical perspective, providing a distinct set of physical and mental advantages. Examine the transforming properties of key inversion asanas:

1. Sirsasana (Head Stand):

Headstand, sometimes known as the "king of asanas," increases blood flow to the brain, promoting mental clarity and rejuvenation. It also fortifies the shoulders, arms, and core.

2. Sarvangasana (Shoulderstand): Recognized as the "queen of asanas," this pose stimulates the thyroid gland, improving metabolism and hormone balance. This inversion encourages relaxation, aids digestion, and strengthens the upper body.

3. Adho Mukha Svanasana (Downward-Facing Dog): While not a typical inversion, Downward-Facing Dog is a simple pose that offers the advantages of one. It stretches the hamstrings and spine while strengthening the arms, shoulders and legs.

4. Pincha Mayurasana (Forearm Stand): Improves upper body strength and balance. This inversion promotes playfulness while also improving concentration and focus.

5. Viparita Karani (Legs-Up-the-Wall Pose): This restorative inversion calms the nervous system, relieves tension, and offers a gentle method to reap the advantages of inversions.

6. Halasana (Plow Pose): This pose stretches the spine and shoulders, stimulates abdominal organs, and promotes relaxation. It is commonly used in sequences to prepare for deeper inversions.

7. Handstand (Adho Mukha Vrksasana): This pose strengthens the upper body and core, improves balance, and promotes a sense of empowerment. It demands concentration, courage, and coordination.

Inversions provide a fresh perspective, both physically and mentally. They test the body, increase strength, and promote balance, all while challenging practitioners to overcome fear and develop mental resilience. Incorporating inversions into a yoga practice in "The Yoga Custom" enhances the whole experience.

B. Pranayama, or yoga breath control, involves more than just breathing. It is a profound investigation of the breath's transformational potential, which affects both the physical and mental states. Learn about key pranayama techniques and their benefits:

1. Ujjayi Pranayama (Victorious Breath): This practice involves blowing in and out via the nose while tightening the back of the throat to create a faint sound. This practice improves attention, warms the body, and promotes contemplative states.

2. Nadi Shodhana: Breathing via alternate nostrils balances the brain's two hemispheres. It relaxes the nervous system, lowers tension, and improves mental clarity.

3. Kapalabhati (Skull-Shining Breath): This technique involves exhaling quickly and forcefully, then inhaling passively. This revitalizing procedure clears the respiratory system, boosts oxygen supply, and revitalizes the body.

4. Bhramari Pranayama (Bee Breath): Creating a humming sound during exhale helps quiet the mind and reduce stress. It is especially efficient at calming the neurological system.

5. Dirga Pranayama (Three-Part Breath): Practice deep diaphragmatic breathing to fully expand the lungs. This approach induces relaxation, increases lung capacity, and improves overall respiratory function.

6. Anulom Vilom (Alternate Nostril Breathing Variation): Like Nadi Shodhana, Anulom Vilom requires alternate nostrils. It regulates the flow of prana, increases respiratory efficiency, and promotes mental clarity.

7. Sitali Pranayama (Cooling Breath): Inhaling through a curled tongue or puckered lips produces a cooling sensation. This breath cools down the body, relieves stress, and calms the neurological system.

i.1. Ujjayi Pranayama (Victorious Breath): Inhale deeply through the nose, slightly restricting the throat, and exhale to create a soothing oceanic sound.

Benefits: Improves attention, warms the body, and promotes meditative states.

2. Nadi Shodhana (Alternate Nostril Breathing): Inhale through one nostril, close it with the thumb, then exhale through the other nostril. Repeat.

Benefits: Balances the hemispheres of the brain, soothes the nervous system and improves mental clarity.

3. Kapalabhati (Skull-Shining Breath): Exhale rapidly and forcefully, then inhale passively via the nose.

Benefits: Cleans the respiratory system, boosts oxygen supply, and energizes the body.

4. Bhramari Pranayama (Bee Breath): Inhale deeply and expel with a humming sound like a bee.

Benefits: Relaxes the mind, lowers stress, and soothes the neurological system.

5. Dirga Pranayama (Three-Part Breath): Inhale deeply into the abdomen, extend the ribcage, and fill the chest. Exhale in reverse sequence.

Benefits: Increases relaxation, lung capacity, and respiratory function.

6. Anulom Vilom (Alternate Nostril Breathing Method): Inhale through one nostril, exhale through the other, then swap nostrils for the following cycle.

Benefits: Regulates prana flow, increases respiratory efficiency, and promotes mental clarity.

7. Sitali Pranayama (Cooling Breath): Inhale with a curled tongue or pursed lips and expel via the nose.

Benefits: Cools the body, relieves tension, and calms the nerves.

Pranayama practices are excellent tools for balancing the breath, mind, and body. Within "The Yoga Custom," regular practice cultivates mental clarity, emotional balance, and a greater connection to the present moment in addition to improving physical well-being.

Meditation and Mindfulness: Developing Inner Presence.

1. Mindfulness. Meditation is focusing on the present moment and observing thoughts and sensations objectively. Use your breath as an anchor.

Benefits: Reduces stress, increases self-awareness, and produces a state of calm and clarity.

2. Loving Kindness Meditation (Metta) aims to cultivate love and compassion for oneself and others. Use phrases such, "May I/you be happy, may I/you be healthy."

Benefits: Promotes empathy, compassion, and a cheerful attitude.

3. Body Scan Meditation: This technique involves systematically focusing attention on different sections of the body to promote awareness and calm.

Benefits: Reduces stress, increases physiological awareness, and generates a state of relaxation.

4. Transcendental Meditation (TM): Repeat a mantra silently for 15-20 minutes to transcend cognition.

Benefits: Promotes deep relaxation, lowers tension, and improves mental clarity.

5. Zen Meditation (Zazen) involves sitting in a certain position, focusing on the breath or a koan (question or statement), and observing thoughts objectively.

Benefits: Promotes attention, clarity, and direct encounter with reality.

6. Guided Visualization. Meditation involves following verbal guidance to imagine peaceful images or beneficial experiences that engage the senses.

Benefits: Increases creativity, decreases anxiety and promotes inner calm.

7. Vipassana Meditation Technique: Observe physical sensations with equanimity.

Benefits: Increases insight into the essence of reality, encourages mindfulness, and improves focus.

Meditation and mindfulness techniques in "The Yoga Custom" lead to inner quiet, self-discovery, and a greater awareness of the present moment. Regular use of these practices can lead to significant mental, emotional, and spiritual well-being.

A. Dhyana: cultivating inner stillness.

Dhyana, often known as meditation, is the practice of cultivating inner calm and obtaining a high level of concentrated awareness. Dhyana, according to "The Yoga Custom," is a pathway to self-realization and a deeper connection with one's true essence.

1. Breath Awareness Meditation: The breathing Awareness Meditation technique involves focusing on the natural flow of the breath, monitoring each inhalation and exhale. Allow the breath to become the focus point, anchoring the attention to the present moment.

Benefits: Promotes mindfulness, soothes the mind, and improves focus.

2. Mantra Meditation: Repeat a chosen mantra silently or aloud. Allow the rhythmic repetition to lead the mind to a state of inner calm.

Benefits: Improves attention, promotes relaxation, and facilitates transcendental experiences.

3. Body Scan Meditation: This technique involves systematically focusing attention on different parts of the body to increase awareness and release tension. Allow a sense of presence to pervade every part.

Benefits: Increases body awareness, promotes relaxation, and strengthens the mind-body connection.

4. The Loving Kindness Meditation (Metta) technique involves extending love and compassion to oneself and others. Make remarks like "May I/you be happy, may I/you be healthy" to foster a positive attitude.

Benefits: Develop empathy, a cheerful attitude, and a kind heart.

5. Visualization Meditation Technique: Create vivid mental images that lead the mind through peaceful landscapes or good scenarios. Engage the senses to create a profound inner experience.

Benefits: Increases creativity, decreases stress and promotes inner calm.

6. Mindfulness of Thought Meditation technique: observe thoughts without attachment or judgment. Allow them to arise and die while retaining a detached awareness.

Benefits: Improves brain clarity, minimizes overthinking, and promotes a thoughtful approach to thoughts.

7. Transcendental Meditation (TM): Repeat a mantra silently to transcend normal cognitive processes. Enter a condition of pure consciousness.

Benefits: Promotes deep relaxation, decreases tension, and encourages inner calm.

Dhyana is a transforming technique in "The Yoga Custom" that leads practitioners on a profound inner journey. Regular practice of these meditation techniques can lead to feelings of inner serenity, increased awareness, and a better understanding of oneself.

i.1. Mindfulness Meditation: Mindfulness meditation involves focusing on the present moment and observing thoughts and sensations without attachment. Use your breath as an anchor.

Benefits: Reduces stress, increases self-awareness, and produces a state of calm and clarity.

2. Loving-Kindness Meditation (Metta): The technique involves cultivating feelings of love and compassion.

Benefits: Promotes empathy, compassion, and a cheerful attitude.

3. Body Scan Meditation: Systematically focus on different body regions to increase awareness and relaxation.

Benefits: Reduces stress, increases physiological awareness, and generates a state of relaxation.

4. Transcendental Meditation (TM) involves repeating a certain mantra silently for 15-20 minutes. Allow the mind to move beyond regular cognition.

Benefits: Promotes deep relaxation, lowers tension, and improves mental clarity.

5. Zen Meditation (Zazen): The technique involves sitting in a precise position, focusing on breath or koan, and observing ideas without attachment.

Benefits: Promotes attention, clarity, and direct encounter with reality.

6. Guided Visualization Meditation: Follow verbal prompts to envision peaceful scenes or positive experiences.

Benefits: Increases creativity, decreases anxiety and promotes inner calm.

7. Vipassana Meditation Technique: Observe physical sensations with equanimity.

Benefits: Increases insight into the essence of reality, encourages mindfulness, and improves focus.

8. Breath Awareness Meditation: Observe each inhale and expiration.

Benefits: Promotes mindfulness, soothes the mind, and improves focus.

9. Mantra Meditation: Repeat a chosen mantra silently or aloud. Allow the rhythmic repetition to lead the mind into quiet.

Benefits: Improves attention, promotes relaxation, and enables transcendental experiences.

10. Visualizations The Meditation technique involves visualizing peaceful environments or pleasant scenarios.

Benefits: Increases creativity, decreases stress and promotes inner calm.

Each meditation practice takes a unique approach to developing mindfulness, inner calm, and self-awareness. Experiment with several ways to see what best fits your particular path within "The Yoga Custom."

ii. Incorporating Mindfulness into Daily Life with "The Yoga Custom":

1. Practice mindful breathing throughout your day. Whether you're in a conference, commuting, or at home, a few focused breaths can help you return to the present moment.

2. Mindful Eating: Enjoy every bite during meals. Pay attention to the tastes, textures, and experiences. Eating mindfully helps you connect with the nourishment your meal gives.

3. Practice mindful walking by paying attention to each step. Feel the earth beneath you, take in your surroundings, and let your movements become a type of meditation.

4. Mindful Work: Complete activities with complete concentration. Whether you're responding to emails, working on a project, or attending meetings, stay focused on the task at hand.

5. Mindful Listening: Actively listen during conversations. Give your whole attention to the speaker and don't plan your response. This promotes deeper connections and understanding.

6. Take small attentive stops throughout the day. Close your eyes, take deep breaths and center yourself. These periods of stillness might help to refuel and concentrate your mind.

7. Mindful Technology Use: Consciously interact with technology. Set screen time limits, prevent multitasking, and be mindful of how digital interactions affect your well-being.

8. Mindful Reflection: Before sleeping, review your day without judgment. Acknowledge your experiences, show thanks, and let go of any remaining tension.

9. Practice Mindful Interactions: Be nice and present during interactions. Whether with family, friends, or colleagues, be present in the moment to develop lasting connections.

10. Mindful Appreciation: Appreciate the beauty around you. It might be the warmth of the sun, the rustle of

leaves, or the taste of your morning coffee. Mindful appreciation improves your connection to the present.

Integrating mindfulness into daily life within "The Yoga Custom" results in a fundamental shift in how you perceive and interact with the environment. These mindful practices promote a sense of presence, gratitude, and a deeper connection to the richness of the present moment.

Adopting a Yogic Lifestyle with "The Yoga Custom":

1. Ahimsa (Non-Violence): Develop compassion and kindness for oneself and others. Choose behaviors, ideas, and words that foster harmony while avoiding damage.

2. Satya (Truthfulness): Be honest in all phases of life. Be true to your words, actions, and thoughts to promote authenticity and integrity.

3. Asteya (Non-Stealing): Show respect for others' assets and ideas. Cultivate contentment with what you have and avoid desiring or taking what isn't yours.

4. Brahmacharya (Moderation): Maintain moderation in all aspects of life, including eating, labor, and leisure. Find a balance to save energy for spiritual growth.

5. Aparigraha (Non-Attachment): Let go of material attachments and cultivate detachment. Accept simplicity and recognize the impermanence of material riches.

6. Saucha (Cleanliness): Ensure cleanliness in both your physical surroundings and personal hygiene. A clean environment promotes clear and concentrated thinking.

7. Santosha (satisfaction): Cultivate satisfaction with life's experiences. Accept thankfulness for the present moment and avoid concentrating on the need for more.

8. Tapas (Self-Discipline): Practice self-discipline in your daily routine, including yoga. Consistent effort and dedication result in spiritual progress.

9. Svadhyaya (Self-Study): Promote self-reflection and study. Explore your inner ideas, feelings, and motives to promote personal growth.

10. Ishvara Pranidhana (Surrender to a Higher Power): Submit your ego and wants to a greater purpose. Develop humility and recognize the interconnection of all beings.

By accepting these yogic concepts in "The Yoga Custom," you not only improve your physical health but also lay the groundwork for spiritual progress. A yogic lifestyle goes beyond the mat, helping you to a more balanced, aware, and purposeful way of life.

A. Living a Sattvic Lifestyle with "The Yoga Custom":

1. Sattvic Diet: Eat fresh, organic fruits and vegetables. Avoid processed foods and develop attentive eating habits. Prioritize purity and simplicity in your meals.

2. Mindful Consumption: Be aware of what you consume, including food, media, relationships, and activities. Choose inspirations that are uplifting and inspiring.

3. Create a balanced daily routine with time for self-care, work, leisure, and spiritual practice. Create a rhythm that benefits both the body and the mind.

4. Maintain a quiet and clean living space. Arrange your surroundings to promote relaxation, including natural light and soothing colors.

5. Regular exercise enhances strength, flexibility, and well-being. Incorporate yoga poses, nature hikes, or any other type of exercise that appeals to you.

6. Mindfulness Practices: Incorporate mindfulness into your routine. Increase your awareness of the current moment through meditation, breath awareness, or mindful activities.

7. Cultivate Positivity: Encourage positive thinking and attitudes. Practice thankfulness and focus on the good things in your life. Limit your exposure to negativity and create a happy outlook.

8. Foster a connection with nature by spending time outdoors regularly. Connect with the natural world to cultivate a sense of balance, whether through a walk in the park, gardening, or simply enjoying the great outdoors.

9. Practice regular self-reflection. Evaluate your thoughts, actions, and intentions. Cultivate self-awareness to match your life with higher values.

10. Service to Others: Exercise seva, or selfless service to benefit others. Perform acts of kindness and positively contribute to your community, instilling a sense of connectivity.

Living a Sattvic lifestyle under "The Yoga Custom" entails building an environment and mindset that is consistent with purity, harmony, and balance.

Incorporating these techniques into your daily routine promotes physical health, mental clarity, and spiritual growth.

i.1. Follow a Sattvic diet that includes organic fruits and vegetables, whole grains, nuts, seeds, and dairy. Avoid processed foods, stimulants, and extremely hot or heavy meals.

2. Mindful Eating: Enjoy each bite, chew properly, and pay attention to hunger and fullness signs. Make your dining area a relaxing place.

3. Stay hydrated with fresh water throughout the day. Hydration promotes biological functioning, assists digestion, and improves general well-being.

4. Practice moderation in food intake. Avoid overeating and instead aim for a well-balanced, varied diet rich in important nutrients.

5. Use seasonal and locally sourced foods whenever possible. Fresh, seasonal produce not only benefits the environment but also meets the body's natural demands.

6. Ayurvedic Principles: Understand your constitution (dosha) and make food choices that promote balance and harmony in body and mind.

7. Plant-Based Protein Options: Include lentils, tofu, and tempeh. Consider plant-based meals for better digestion and general wellness.

8. Pre and post-yoga nutrition: Prefer light, easily digestible snacks like fruits or smoothies. After practice,

eat a balanced supper that includes carbohydrates, proteins, and healthy fats.

9. Mind-Body Connection: Become aware of how different nutrients impact your energy, mood, and overall well-being. Pay attention to your body's messages regarding dietary choices.

10. Practice intuitive eating by listening to your body's hunger and fullness cues. Eat when hungry and quit when full, promoting a positive connection with food.

Nutrition and diet are viewed in "The Yoga Custom" not only as a means of nourishing the body but also as a way to promote overall well-being and improve yoga practice. By making deliberate and thoughtful decisions, you can match your food with the principles of balance, harmony, and vitality.

ii. Balancing Your Daily Routine at "The Yoga Custom":

1. Morning Ritual: Begin the day with gratitude and positive goals. To awaken your body and mind, use techniques such as meditation, breathing exercises, or moderate stretches.

2. Yoga Asana Practice: Make time for your yoga asana practice, whether it's a complete sequence or a few core postures. This helps to align your body, increase flexibility, and promote mindfulness.

3. Mindful Breakfast: Incorporate Sattvic foods for a wholesome and mindful breakfast experience. Spend time savoring each bite, cultivating a mindful approach to your first meal of the day.

4. Focus on the job or daily responsibilities to maximize productivity. Time management and work prioritization can help you feel accomplished.

5. Mindful Breaks: Take brief breaks throughout the day. To recharge your energy and calm your thoughts, use these moments to practice mindful breathing, stretching, or a short stroll.

6. Nourishing Lunch: Incorporate a diverse range of meals for a balanced and nutritious lunch. Avoid rushing and establish a relaxing atmosphere for your midday meal.

7. Set aside time for creative or learning activities. Encourage creativity and constant learning through activities such as reading, writing, drawing, and hobbies.

8. Nature Connection: Explore the outdoors and connect with nature. This could include taking a walk in the park, gardening, or simply appreciating the natural surroundings to recharge your spirit.

9. Afternoon Recharge: Take a little break in the afternoon to unwind. Consider practicing meditation, deep breathing, or taking a short nap to restore your energy for the rest of the day.

10. Evening Reflection: End your day with a time of reflection. Review your accomplishments, express thanks, and identify areas for improvement. This prepares your thoughts for a relaxing evening.

11. Evening Yoga or Stretching: Practice easy yoga or stretching to relieve tension from the day. This activity gets your body ready for a good night's sleep.

12. Mindful Dinner: Eat simply and mindfully, avoiding heavy or stimulating foods close to bedtime. Create a relaxing setting for your evening meal.

13. Establish a relaxing evening ritual, such as reading, meditation, or light relaxation activities. This indicates to your body and mind that it is time to relax.

14. Quality Sleep: Ensure ample and quality sleep. Create a sleep-friendly environment and stick to a consistent sleep pattern to improve overall health.

By creating a balanced daily practice in "The Yoga Custom," you can combine your physical, mental, and spiritual elements. Each part contributes to a comprehensive strategy that promotes a sense of purpose, balance, and mindfulness in your daily life.

Exploring the Spiritual Dimension of "The Yoga Custom":

1. Meditation Practice: Establish a regular meditation practice to explore your inner self. Explore several meditation techniques to see what resonates with your spiritual path.

2. Mindful Awareness: Practice mindful awareness throughout the day. Encourage a stronger sense of presence and connection during activities, interactions, and moments of solitude.

3. Self-Reflection: Consider your views, values, and purpose. Assess your spiritual path regularly to encourage ongoing growth and insight.

4. Integrate Sacred Rituals into Your Routine. This could include morning rituals, prayers, or ceremonies that reflect your spiritual views and instill a sense of sacredness.

5. Connect with the Divine: Establish a personal connection with a higher power that speaks to you. This could include prayer, devotion, or acts that promote a sense of spiritual connectedness.

6. Study Sacred writings: Find writings or philosophical teachings that align with your spiritual journey. Dive into the knowledge of ancient cultures to gain a better grasp of spirituality.

7. Service and Compassion: Promote selfless service (seva) and compassion for others. Acts of kindness and service improve the spiritual well-being of both the giver and the receiver.

8. Nature as a Teacher: Connect with nature for spiritual inspiration. Nature can be a powerful teacher, whether through hikes in natural settings, gardening, or simply enjoying the beauty of the outdoors.

9. Community Connection: Connect with a spiritual community or like-minded people. Share your spiritual experiences, thoughts, and practices to help you feel connected and supported.

10. Yoga Philosophy: Analyze the philosophical components of yoga. Explore ideas such as the interconnection of all beings, the nature of awareness, and the path to self-realization.

11. Develop a gratitude practice to appreciate the blessings in your life. Expressing thankfulness strengthens your connection with the divine and promotes a happy attitude.

12. Allow for moments of inner silence throughout the day. These calm moments allow for spiritual introspection and listening to your soul's whispers.

13. Mind-Body Connection: Understand the relationship between mind, body, and spirit. Yoga asanas, pranayama, and holistic well-being are all practices that help with spiritual integration.

14. Lifelong Learning: View your spiritual path as an ongoing learning process. Stay open to new thoughts,

experiences, and viewpoints that can help you grow spiritually.

The spiritual side of "The Yoga Custom" is a deep examination of self-discovery, connection, and transcendence. By adopting these practices into your daily life, you go on a journey to nourish your spiritual essence and expand your perception of the divine inside and around you.

A. Connecting with the Divine through "The Yoga Custom":

1. Prayer and Devotion: Pray with sincerity and devotion. Create a sacred area in which you can connect with the divine through genuine communication.

2. Add meditative reflection to your spiritual practice. Allow for peaceful moments of reflection to foster a stronger relationship with the divine within.

3. Create holy rituals that align with your spiritual views. These rituals, whether they involve lighting candles, conducting ceremonial acts, or following specific traditions, help to establish a palpable connection.

4. Nature as Sacred: Consider nature as a manifestation of the divine. Spend time outside, admiring the natural world's beauty and acknowledging the holiness that exists in all living beings.

5. Incorporate devotional chanting into your practice. This practice creates a heart-centered connection by chanting traditional mantras, hymns, or specific heavenly names.

6. Service to Others: Seeing service to others as a means of connecting with the divine in all beings. Acts of kindness and selflessness become sacred offerings to the heavenly presence.

7. Contemplation of Sacred Texts: Read and reflect on texts relevant to your spiritual development. Allow the knowledge found in these writings to guide your understanding and enhance your connection.

8. Mindful Gratitude: Acknowledge the divine presence in the riches of your life. Express thanks for both obstacles and blessings, realizing that they are all part of a divine plan.

9. Practice silent communication with the divine. Engage in moments of inner silence, listening to your soul's whispers and connecting with the divine presence inside.

10. Ceremonial Offerings: Create offerings to express your commitment. These contributions could be actual or symbolic demonstrations of your devotion and reverence.

11. Inner Dialogue: Establish an ongoing dialogue with the divine. Develop a state of openness and receptivity, allowing guidance and insight to enter your consciousness.

12. Sacred Arts and Creativity:

Sacred art or creative efforts allow you to express your relationship to the divine. Allow your art to be a source of devotion and heavenly inspiration.

13. Community Connection: Participate in spiritual communities with those who share your beliefs. Shared activities, rituals, and group dedication heighten the feeling of spiritual connection.

14. Gracious Acceptance: Embrace life's flow as divine unfolding. Embrace both obstacles and successes as chances for spiritual growth.

Connecting with the divine in "The Yoga Custom" is an intensely intimate and transforming experience. Through these practices, you open doors to experiencing the sacred in all aspects of your life, cultivating a deep sense of connection and union with the divine essence.

i. Explore Bhakti Yoga in "The Yoga Custom":

1. Engage in devotional rituals, such as prayer, chanting, and singing bhajans, to show love and devotion to the divine.

2. Practice surrender and trust in the divine. Release attachments by understanding that every event is part of a divine plan for your spiritual development.

3. Engage in worship and rituals that align with your spiritual journey. Create a sacred space for divine contact through ritual practices.

4. Bhakti Mantras: Incorporate them into your daily practice. Chanting sacred names and chants activates the divine presence and strengthens your connection.

5. Develop love and compassion in all areas of life. Embodying these attributes reflects the core of Bhakti Yoga and promotes a heart-centered way of living.

6. Seva (Selfless Service): Express your devotion to the divine by performing selfless acts. Acts of kindness and service become a type of devotion and a gift to the almighty.

7. Bhakti Philosophy: Understand the philosophy of Bhakti yoga. Explore writings and teachings that stress the path of love and dedication to gain a deeper understanding of this transforming practice.

8. Establish a personal and intimate relationship with the Divine. Create a sense of connection that extends beyond ceremonial behaviors, allowing for direct and emotional communication.

9. Use religious imagery or symbols that align with your dedication. Icons, images, or symbols of the divine can serve as focal points for your spiritual activities.

10. Reverence for All Beings: Love and respect all beings. Recognize the divine presence in others, cultivating a sense of unity and compassion through your encounters.

11. Demonstrate thankfulness and humility as displays of devotion. Recognize the divine grace in all aspects of your life and cultivate a thankful attitude.

12. Consider Attending Devotional Retreats or Gatherings. Being in the presence of like-minded people can boost the collective energy of dedication and improve your spiritual experience.

13. Engage in inner discourse with the Divine. Communicate your ideas, feelings, and goals with openness and receptivity.

14. Incorporate Bhakti Yoga into your daily life. Allow your actions, ideas, and interactions to be led by the spirit of love, dedication, and reverence to the divine.

Bhakti Yoga is described in "The Yoga Custom" as a path of intense love and devotion. These practices develop a heart-centered connection with the divine, resulting in a transformative path toward spiritual awakening.

ii. Explore Karma Yoga in "The Yoga Custom":

1. Embrace Selfless Service (Seva) as a Spiritual Practice. Engage in actions without regard for the outcome, offering your efforts for the benefit of others.

2. Mindful activity: Perform each activity with complete awareness. Approach each moment as an opportunity for spiritual growth, whether at work, in relationships, or daily.

3. Develop detachment from the outcomes of your activities. Concentrate on the process and aim rather than being overly preoccupied about success or failure.

4. Compassionate Engagement: Practice compassion in your interactions. Extend love and understanding, acknowledging the interdependence of all beings in the chain of karma.

5. Align your behaviors with your dharma (righteous responsibility). Identify your obligations in various roles and endeavor to carry them out with integrity and sincerity.

6. labor as Worship: Consider your labor a kind of worship. Dedicate your efforts to a greater purpose, realizing that any activity can be spiritually significant.

7. Surrender the results of your deeds to the divine. Recognize that you are just an instrument, and the results are part of a broader cosmic plan.

8. Maintain non-attachment to the ego. Let go of personal desires and egoic identification, acknowledging the illusion of a separate self within the magnificent fabric of reality.

9. Balanced Living: Strive for a healthy balance of activities and rest. Avoid overexertion and understand the value of self-care in maintaining your ability to give selflessly.

10. Mindful Decision-Making: Think about how your decision will affect others and the larger context. Strive for decisions that are consistent with the values of righteousness and harmony.

11. Practice thankfulness through your deeds. Recognize the possibilities and resources that are available to you, and demonstrate thanks via your focused efforts.

12. Make a positive contribution to your community. Seek opportunities to help and uplift those around you, understanding that communal well-being is inextricably linked with individual acts.

13. Develop an awareness of connectivity among all beings. Recognize that your activities reverberate

through the fabric of existence, influencing collective karma.

14. Continuous Learning: Treat life as an ongoing learning process. Learn from every event, viewing both problems and accomplishments as chances for personal development on the Karma Yoga path.

Karma Yoga is described in "The Yoga Custom" as a transformational path of selfless service and attentive action. By accepting these principles, you create a tapestry of positive karma, which benefits both your spiritual progress and the well-being of the world around you.

Integrating Yoga into Modern Life: "The Yoga Custom"

1. Mindful Morning Routine: Begin each day with mindfulness. To start the day off well, try mild stretches, aware breathing, or a brief meditation.

2. Yoga Breaks at Work: Take small yoga breaks throughout the day. To refresh your mind and body, try easy stretches, deep breathing exercises, or brief mindfulness activities.

3. Desk Yoga: Practice desk-friendly yoga positions. Stretch your neck, shoulders, and spine to relieve tension and improve posture, increasing overall health during sedentary work hours.

4. Mindful Eating: Practice mindful eating. Pay attention to your meals, relish each bite, and create a bond between your body and the sustenance it receives.

5. Yoga Nidra for Relaxation: Use guided relaxation to relieve tension. Short sessions during breaks or before bedtime can help promote relaxation and improved sleep.

6. Create a Tech-Free Wind Down Routine. Disconnect from electronics at least an hour before bedtime and engage in relaxing activities like mild yoga, reading, or meditation.

7. Yoga for Commuting: Make your commute a thoughtful experience. Deep breathing, listening to relaxing music, or engaging in mindfulness exercises might help you stay centered during your drive.

8. Family Yoga Time: Engage the entire family in yoga activities. Practice easy yoga positions or meditation together to develop a sense of well-being and community.

9. Mindful Walking: Practice mindfulness during your walks. Pay attention to your breath, the sensation of movement, and the surroundings as you transform a typical activity into a meditation exercise.

10. Plan periodic digital detox yoga retreats. Unplug from technology, practice yoga, and reconnect with nature to recharge your mind, body, and spirit.

11. Yoga for difficult Moments: Create a collection of brief yoga practices for difficult situations. Deep breathing exercises, grounding positions, or a few moments of mindfulness can bring immediate comfort.

12. Online Yoga sessions: Try online yoga sessions to improve flexibility. Incorporate virtual courses into your daily routine to gain access to a variety of styles and teachings, making yoga more accessible to those with hectic schedules.

13. Yoga Challenges with Friends: Participate in yoga challenges with your friends or colleagues. Set common goals, discuss progress, and build a supportive community around your yoga practice.

14. introspective Journaling: Integrate yoga with introspective journaling. Write about your experiences, insights, and feelings after yoga sessions to promote self-awareness and personal development.

By incorporating yoga into modern life as part of "The Yoga Custom," you not only improve your physical health but also create mindfulness, resilience, and a sense of balance in the face of modern-day challenges.

A. Practice Yoga Off the Mat in "The Yoga Custom":

1. Mindful Breathing in Daily Life: Incorporate mindful breathing into your daily activities. Whether you're commuting, working, or waiting in line, take deliberate breaths to keep focused and relaxed.

2. Cultivate Present Moment Awareness. Engage fully in tasks, discussions, and experiences without being distracted by past regrets or future concerns.

3. Integrating Yoga Philosophy: Use yoga philosophy to tackle daily issues. Accept concepts such as nonattachment, compassion, and mindfulness as guiding principles in decision-making and interactions.

4. Appreciation Practice: Incorporate appreciation into your daily routine. Take time to appreciate the little delights of life, which will help you develop a positive outlook and a stronger connection to the richness of life.

5. Conscious Eating: Practice mindful eating. Be mindful of the flavors, textures, and nutrients in each bite. Eating thoughtfully improves your connection to food and its impact on your health.

6. Mindful Technology Use: Be mindful when using technology. Set screen time limits, prevent multitasking, and be deliberate about your online interactions to avoid unneeded stress and distraction.

7. Compassionate Communication: Promote compassionate communication. Be conscious of your words, listen actively, and express yourself with kindness to promote healthy relationships in all aspects of life.

8. Emotional Regulation: Practice yoga for emotional regulation. When presented with a hardship, use deep breathing, meditation, or grounding practices to negotiate your emotions with awareness and resilience.

9. Service for Others: Provide unselfish service beyond the mat. Look for ways to give back to your community by helping others with kindness and charity.

10. Staying Grounded in Chaos: Maintain a sense of stability throughout turbulent settings. In times of stress or uncertainty, mentally perform grounding positions to promote stability and inner serenity.

11. Practice intuitive decision-making. Trust your inner direction and connect with your intuition to create choices that are true to your actual self.

12. Cultivating Stillness in Action: Practice stillness in action. Even amid a hectic day, seek moments of inner peace and tranquility to promote mental clarity and attention.

13. giving and Giving: Develop a spirit of giving. Share your time, resources, and abilities with others, following the yogic ideal of selfless giving.

14. Mindful Reflection: Add mindful reflection to your routine. Regularly evaluate your ideas, actions, and

aspirations to promote self-awareness and ongoing personal development.

Practicing yoga off the mat in "The Yoga Custom" entails incorporating the essence of yoga into all aspects of your life. By incorporating these concepts, you can develop a comprehensive and transformative approach to living that is consistent with the essential teachings of yoga.

i. Nurturing Relationships using Yoga Principles in "The Yoga Custom":

1. Compassionate Communication: Practice compassionate communication. Listen actively, talk from the heart, and cultivate understanding to promote happy relationships.

2. Practice non-attachment in relationships. Allow for individual development and avoid sticking to expectations, promoting freedom and acceptance.

3. Mindful Presence: Stay fully present in interactions. Practice attentive presence with family, friends, or coworkers to strengthen relationships and understanding.

4. Develop empathy and understanding. Consider others' viewpoints, acknowledge them, and respond with respect and compassion.

5. Yoga for Couples: Enjoy partner yoga as a bonding experience. Participating in yoga together not only improves physical health but also fosters connection and mutual support.

6. Breath Awareness in Conflict: Use breath awareness during disputes. When tensions rise, take thoughtful breaths to relax the nervous system and promote clarity and efficient communication.

7. thankfulness in interactions: Show thankfulness in your interactions. Recognize and appreciate the positive qualities of your relationships, so establish a happy environment.

8. Shared Mindfulness Practices: Incorporate mindfulness into your relationships. Whether through meditation, mindful walks, or cooperative activities, shared awareness fosters connection and mutual progress.

9. Integrate yogic principles into relationships. Accept ideas like ahimsa (nonviolence), sincerity, and contentment to guide your activities.

10. Demonstrate generosity and love in your interactions. Provide your time, support, and affection freely, cultivating a giving attitude among your connections.

11. Self-Reflection in Relationships: Practice self-reflection during relationships. Regularly evaluate your thoughts, actions, and contributions to promote personal development and self-awareness.

12. Balancing independence and togetherness:

Strike a balance between independence and cooperation. Encourage one another's endeavors while simultaneously enjoying joint activities and experiences.

13. Practice mindful listening. Give your complete attention to the speaker, stop from passing judgment, and make room for open and real conversation.

14. Harmony in Diversity: Encourage diversity in relationships. Appreciate and celebrate differences, acknowledging the value they add to the shared fabric of connectedness.

By implementing these concepts into your relationships as described in "The Yoga Custom," you lay the groundwork for harmony, understanding, and love. Yoga goes beyond the mat, impacting how you interact with others and establishing meaningful connections in every aspect of your life.

ii. Stress Management using Yogic Practices in "The Yoga Custom":

1. Deep Breathing Techniques: Deep breathing exercises, such as diaphragmatic or alternate nostril breathing (Nadi Shodhana), can help relax the nervous system and reduce stress.

2. Mindful Meditation: Add mindful meditation to your schedule. Develop present-moment awareness through methods such as mindfulness meditation or guided relaxation (Yoga Nidra).

3. Yoga Asanas for Stress Relief: Incorporate stress-reducing yoga asanas into your practice. Poses such as Child's Pose, Forward Fold, and Legs Up the Wall can help relieve stress and promote relaxation.

4. Practice progressive muscle relaxation.
Systematically tension and release of various muscle
groups to produce physical and mental calm.

5. Practice daily mindfulness. Bring mindfulness to your
actions, whether eating, walking, or working, to promote
a sense of presence and reduce stress.

6. Nature Connection: Enjoy time in nature. Connecting
with nature, whether through a walk in the park or sitting
by a body of water, can help to relax the mind.

7. Yoga for difficult Moments: Create a list of fast yoga
practices for difficult situations. Incorporate breathing
exercises or easy stretches to relieve tension as
needed.

8. Digital Detox: Take regular digital detox breaks.
Reduce stress by disconnecting from screens and
technology.

9. Self-Compassion Practices: Encourage self-
compassion. During difficult circumstances, treat
yourself with kindness, remembering that stress is a
normal part of life and that you are doing your best.

10. Journaling for tension Relief: - Journaling can help
you release tension. Writing about your ideas, emotions,
and concerns allows you to express yourself and reflect.

11. Mind-Body Relaxation strategies: - Learn about
various strategies for relaxing the body. Biofeedback,
gradual muscle relaxation, and autogenic training are all
effective methods for releasing stress.

12. Yoga Retreats for Stress Relief: - Consider attending yoga retreats aimed at stress alleviation. Immersing yourself in a retreat setting can give you a focused space for rest.

13. Laughter Yoga: - Practice laughter yoga. Engage in things that bring you joy and laughter, as laughter has been shown to reduce stress in both the body and the mind.

14. Focus on healthy sleep hygiene. To improve your overall well-being, stick to a consistent sleep regimen, create a comfortable sleep environment, and practice relaxation techniques before bedtime.

According to "The Yoga Custom," stress management entails a comprehensive strategy that incorporates yogic practices, mindfulness, and self-care measures. Incorporating these practices throughout your everyday routine establishes a foundation for resilience, balance, and overall well-being.

Conclusion

In "The Yoga Custom," we see a comprehensive approach to well-being that goes far beyond the confines of a yoga mat. This custom welcomes a transforming journey, beginning with the fundamentals of yoga philosophy and ending with the integration of timeless concepts into current living. The journey begins with self-discovery on the mat, using mindfulness, breath, and movement. It progresses to an exploration of yoga's philosophical underpinnings, introducing us to ancient knowledge and guiding principles. As the practice grows, yoga becomes a way of life, integrated into our everyday routines, relationships, and even stressful circumstances. "The Yoga Custom" highlights the connection between mind, body, and spirit. It teaches us to practice compassion, gratitude, and self-awareness, which promotes both physical flexibility and mental resilience. Yoga extends into our relationships, encouraging us to communicate with love, accept variety, and handle the complexity of modern life with grace. Stress, once a deadly antagonist, is transformed into an opportunity for growth and self-care by yogic practices. From deep breathing to focused meditation, each approach contributes to the tapestry of stress management, creating a haven of peace amid life's problems.

As we end our investigation of "The Yoga Custom," we know that yoga is a journey rather than a destination. A journey that involves continual study, self-reflection, and a commitment to living by the yoga principles. Whether on or off the mat, "The Yoga Custom" is a constantly growing guide, enabling us to discover, adapt, and

accept yoga's transformational power in all aspects of
our lives.

"Welcoming The Yoga Custom: A Multidisciplinary Approach to Well-Being"

In the complex tapestry of life, "The Yoga Custom"
emerges as a guiding philosophy, providing a
comprehensive approach to well-being. This custom,
based on ancient yogic teachings, goes beyond the
limitations of physical practice to become a transforming
journey that touches all aspects of our existence.

Foundations for Self-Discovery:

"The Yoga Custom" is really about self-discovery.
Individuals can achieve physical and mental flexibility by
engaging in mindful movement, breathing, and
contemplation on the mat. The practice becomes a
haven for self-awareness, cultivating a strong bond with
one's own body and mind. "The Yoga Custom" explores
yoga's philosophical roots and everlasting principles.
Ahimsa (nonviolence), Satya (truthfulness), and
santosha (contentment) help practitioners live a
balanced and purposeful life, influencing how they deal
with problems and appreciate moments of delight.

Integration with Modern Life:

The essential core of this custom is its perfect
incorporation into contemporary life. Whether it's a
mindful morning routine, yoga breaks at work, or a
digital detox, "The Yoga Custom" goes beyond the mat
to instill mindfulness and purpose in daily activities. It
becomes a companion in the rush and bustle, providing

moments of calm amidst the mayhem. "The Yoga Custom" promotes compassionate communication, non-attachment, and empathy to balance relationships. It becomes a guiding force in building partnerships based on love, understanding, and mutual progress. Partner yoga and mindfulness activities help to enhance the bonds of togetherness. Stress can be transformed into an opportunity for progress through "The Yoga Custom." Breath awareness, mindful meditation, and laughter yoga help people develop resilience and find shelter in the present moment, fostering a sense of serenity even in the face of life's obstacles.

Conclusion: A Lifelong Journey of Transformation

To summarize, "Embracing the Yoga Custom: A Holistic Approach to Well-Being" is more than just a practice; it is a lifelong adventure. It's a journey that connects ancient knowledge, modern adaptation, and personal growth. Whether on the mat, in relationships, or managing stress, "The Yoga Custom" serves as a constant guide, enabling people to embrace yoga's transforming power in all aspects of their lives.